The Ultimate Instant Pot Fish Recipes

Easy, Hands-Off Recipes for Your Instant Pot

Michelle Adriani

Sommario

Introduction 5

Fish and Seafood 7

Lime Octopus 7

Garlic Cuttlefish 9

Calamari in Pepper Sauce 12

Paprika and Rosemary Salmon 14

Chile Fish Curry 16

Seafood Paella 18

Soybeans and Cod Stew 20

Salmon Pie 23

Mackerel Patties 26

Oregano Whitebait 28

Rosemary Mackerel Salad 30

Monkfish Wine Stew 32

Eggplant Cod Chowder 34

Salmon Mustard Tacos 37

Sriracha Shrimp 40

Tuna Noodles Salad 42

Oregano Snapper 44

Garlic Mussel Soup 46

Doughy Salmon Bars 48

Halibut with Ginger Sauce 50

Snapper with Onions 53

Coconut Cod 56

Sweet Creamy Mackerel 58

Chili Anchovy..60

Marinated Shrimps...62

Shrimp Lemon Cocktail..65

Cheddar Mussels Casserole...67

Ricotta Shrimps..69

Butter Scallops...72

Cajun Crab Casserole...74

Crab Melt with Monterey Jack..76

Lemongrass Baked Snapper...78

Salmon Onion Salad...80

Cod Loin...82

Salmon in Cream Sauce...84

Kohlrabi Gratin with Salmon..86

Zucchini Mussel Chowder..88

Turmeric Salmon Skewers...90

ProvoloneTuscan Shrimps...92

Garlic Parmesan Scallops..94

Seafood Bisque..96

Lobster Bisque...98

Lemon Lobster...100

Milky Mussels...102

Tuna Egg Cakes..104

Salmon under Parmesan..106

Salmon Poppers...109

Tuna Nutmeg Rolls...111

Tilapia Sticks..114

Rangoon Crab Dip 116

Conclusion..119

Introduction

This complete and also useful guide to instant pot food preparation with over 1000 dishes for morning meal, supper, supper, and also treats! This is one of the most detailed split second pot recipe books ever published thanks to its range and also accurate guidelines. Innovative dishes as well as classics, modern-day take on household's most enjoyed meals-- all this is delicious, simple and of course as healthy as it can be. Change the way you cook with these ingenious split second pot guidelines. Need a new dinner or a treat? Here you are! Best immediate pot meals integrated in a couple of basic actions, also a novice can do it! The instant pot defines the means you prepare everyday. This instant pot recipe book aids you make the absolute most out of your regular food selection.

The only split second pot book you will ever before require with the supreme collection of recipes will help you in the direction of an easier as well as much healthier cooking area experience. If you want to conserve time cooking meals extra successfully, if you want to provide your family food that can satisfy even the pickiest eater, you remain in the best location! Master your split second pot and also make your cooking needs suit your busy way of life.

Fish and Seafood

Lime Octopus

Prep time: 5 minutes

Cooking time: 15 minutes

Servings: 6

Ingredients:

- 1 teaspoon salt
- 10 ounces octopus
- 1 teaspoon cilantro
- 2 tablespoons olive oil
- 1 teaspoon garlic powder
- 1 teaspoon lime juice
- 1cup of water

Directions:

1. Place the octopus into the pressure cooker.

2. Sprinkle it with the cilantro, garlic powder, and salt and mix well. Add the water into the pressure cooker and close the lid.

3. Set the pressure cooker to "Pressure" mode. Cook the dish on for 8 minutes. Remove the dish from the pressure cooker and put in the tray filled with the octopus.

4. Sprinkle the seafood with olive oil.

5. Preheat the oven to 360 F and transfer the tray to the oven. Cook the dish for 7 minutes.

6. When the octopus is cooked, remove it from the oven and sprinkle with lemon juice. Let it rest briefly before serving.

Nutrition: calories 80, fat 5, fiber 0, carbs 1.49, protein 7

Garlic Cuttlefish

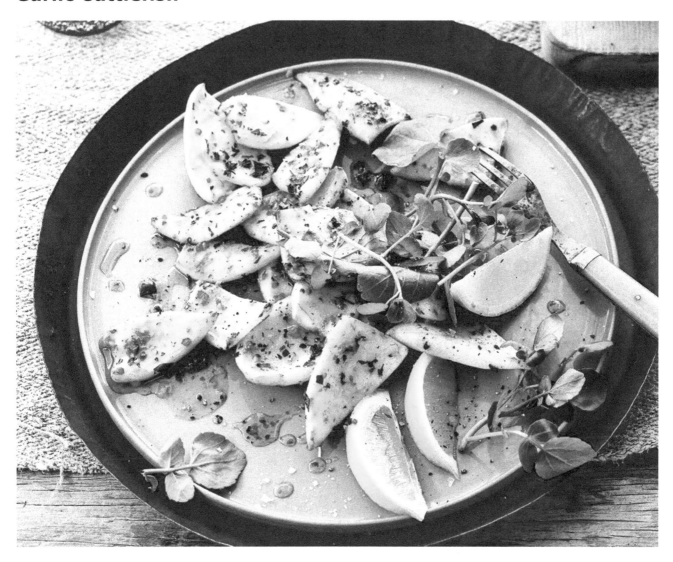

Prep time: 20 minutes

Cooking time: 13 minutes

Servings: 6

Ingredients:

- 1 pound squid
- 1 tablespoon minced garlic
- 1 teaspoon onion powder
- 1 tablespoon lemon juice
- 1 tablespoon chives
- 1 teaspoon salt
- 1 teaspoon white pepper
- 3 tablespoons fish sauce
- 2 tablespoons butter
- ¼ chile pepper

Directions:

1. Slice the squid. Combine the minced garlic, onion powder, chives, salt, and white pepper together in a mixing bowl and stir well and stir.

2. Chop the chile pepper and add it to the spice mixture. Combine the sliced squid and spice mixture together, stirring well.

3. Sprinkle the seafood mixture with the lemon juice and fish sauce and stir. Let the mixture rest for 10 minutes.

4. Set the pressure cooker to "Sauté" mode. Add the butter into the pressure cooker and melt it.

5. Place the sliced squid mixture into the pressure cooker and close the lid. Cook the dish for 13 minutes.

6. When the dish is cooked, remove the food from the pressure cooker. Sprinkle the dish with the liquid from the cooked squid and serve.

Nutrition: calories 112, fat 4.9, fiber 0, carbs 3.92, protein 12

Calamari in Pepper Sauce

Prep time: 10 minutes

Cooking time: 13 minutes

Servings: 4

Ingredients:

- 12 ounces calamari
- 1 white onion
- 1 teaspoon cilantro
- 3 garlic cloves
- 1 teaspoon ground ginger
- ¼ cup fish stock
- 1 teaspoon fresh thyme
- ¼ cup wine
- ¼ cup of water
- 1 tablespoon olive oil
- 3 medium tomatoes
- ½ teaspoon ground white pepper
- 1 teaspoon lime juice

Directions:

1. Wash the calamari carefully and peel it.

2. Slice the calamari into medium-thick slices. Slice the garlic cloves, dice the onion, and c. hop the fresh thyme and tomatoes.

3. Set the pressure cooker to "Sauté" mode.

4. Put the sliced calamari into the pressure cooker and sprinkle it with the olive oil. Sauté the dish for 5 minutes.

5. Add the garlic, onion, thyme, and tomatoes to the pressure cooker.

6. Sprinkle the dish with the water, wine, ground ginger, lime juice, and fish stock, stir well, and close the lid.

7. Set the pressure cooker to "Sauté" mode. Stew the dish for 8 minutes.

8. Remove the cooked calamari from the pressure cooker. Serve the dish hot.

Nutrition: calories 238, fat 6.1, fiber 2, carbs 16.64, protein 29

Paprika and Rosemary Salmon

Prep time: 10 minutes

Cooking time: 15 minutes

Servings: 6

Ingredients:

- 1 pound salmon fillet
- 1 tablespoon marjoram
- ½ teaspoon rosemary
- 1 tablespoons salt
- ½ cup dill
- 1 cup of water
- 1 teaspoon cilantro
- 1 tablespoon paprika
- 1 teaspoon butter
- 1 teaspoon onion powder

Directions:

1. Combine the marjoram, rosemary, and salt in a small bowl.

2. Rub the salmon fillet with the spice mixture.

3. Chop the dill and combine it with the onion powder and paprika in a mixing bowl. Add cilantro and stir well.

4. Place the salmon fillet on the steamer rack and transfer it to the pressure cooker. Set the pressure cooker to "Steam" mode.

5. Sprinkle the salmon with the dill mixture.

6. Close the pressure cooker and cook the fish for 15 minutes.

7. When the cooking time ends, release the remaining pressure and let the salmon rest briefly.

8. Transfer the dish to a serving plate.

Nutrition: calories 127, fat 6.2, fiber 1, carbs 1.17, protein 16

Chile Fish Curry

Prep time: 10 minutes

Cooking time: 10 minutes

Servings: 5

Ingredients:

- 1 tablespoon curry paste
- 1 teaspoon curry
- 1 cup cream
- 1 pound salmon fillet
- ¼ cup garlic clove
- ½ tablespoon salt
- 1 teaspoon cilantro
- ¼ cup of fish sauce
- ½ cup of water
- 1 onion
- 1 teaspoon red chile flakes
- 1 tablespoon fresh ginger

Directions:

1. Chop the salmon fillet roughly and transfer it to the pressure cooker.

2. Combine the cream and fish sauce in a mixing bowl. Sprinkle the liquid mixture with the curry paste and curry and blend until smooth.

3. Peel the garlic cloves and onion.

4. Chop the vegetables and add them to the cream mixture.

5. Grate the ginger and add the ginger, chili flakes, water, salt, and cilantro and mix well. Pour it onto the chopped salmon and coat the fish well.

6. Add the curried fish to the pressure cooker. Close the lid and set the pressure cooker mode to "Pressure."

7. Cook the dish for 10 minutes. When the cooking time ends, release the remaining pressure and open the lid.

8. Transfer the dish to serving bowls.

Nutrition: calories 264, fat 16.2, fiber 2, carbs 7.99, protein 22

Seafood Paella

Prep time: 10 minutes

Cooking time: 15 minutes

Servings: 5

Ingredients:

- 1 cup cauliflower rice
- 8 ounces shrimp
- 5 ounces mussels
- 2 cups fish stock
- 1 cup of water
- 1 tablespoon of sea salt
- 1 small chile pepper
- 1 teaspoon curry
- 1 teaspoon turmeric
- 1 tablespoon oregano
- 1 tablespoon fish sauce
- 1 teaspoon paprika
- 3 garlic cloves

- 1 tablespoon butter

Directions:

1. Peel the shrimp and combine them with the mussels. Place the seafood into the pressure cooker.

2. Add cauliflower rice, salt, curry, turmeric, oregano, and paprika and stir well.

3. Combine the fish stock, fish sauce, and butter together in a mixing bowl and blend well. Pour water mixture into the pressure cooker.

4. Peel the garlic and slice it. Chop the chile pepper.

5. Sprinkle the cauliflower rice mixture with the sliced garlic and chopped chile pepper. Stir briefly using a wooden spoon.

6. Close the pressure cooker lid and set the pressure cooker mode to "Steam". Cook for 15 minutes.

7. When the dish is cooked, remove the food from the pressure cooker. Transfer the paella to a serving bowl.

Nutrition: calories 130, fat 4.7, fiber 1.3, carbs 4.9, protein 16.8

Soybeans and Cod Stew

Prep time: 15 minutes

Cooking time: 30 minutes

Servings: 8

Ingredients:

- 1 pound cod
- 1 large onion
- ¼ cup garlic cloves
- 3 red bell peppers
- 1 teaspoon cilantro
- 1 tablespoon oregano
- 1 teaspoon turmeric
- 4 cups chicken stock
- 1 cup black soybeans, canned
- 1 teaspoon of sea salt
- ¼ cup of fish sauce
- ½ cup of water
- 1 teaspoon red chile flakes

- 1 tablespoon fresh ginger

- ½ cup parsley

- 1 tablespoon ground black pepper

- 1 teaspoon white pepper

Directions:

1. Chop the cod roughly and add it to a mixing bowl.

2. Peel the onion and garlic cloves and dice them and add to the cod.

3. Combine the cilantro, turmeric, sea salt, chili flakes, ground black pepper, and white pepper together in a separate bowl and mix well and stir well.

4. Add the spice mixture to the cod. Add the canned black soybeans and ginger. Chop the parsley.

5. Transfer the cod mixture into the pressure cooker.

6. Add the chicken stock, water, and fish sauce. Sprinkle the stew mixture with the chopped parsley.

7. Stir the stew mixture using a wooden spoon and close the lid. Set the pressure cooker to "Sauté" mode.

8. Cook the dish on for 30 minutes. When the stew is cooked, let it cool briefly and serve.

Nutrition: calories 203, fat 2.2, fiber 5, carbs 27.8, protein 19

Salmon Pie

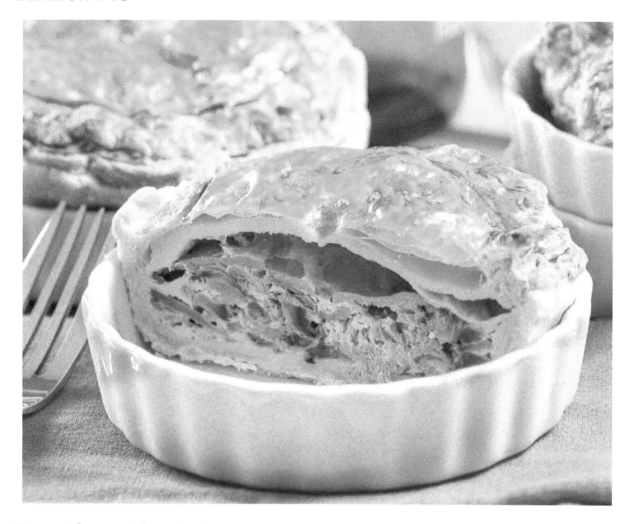

Prep time: 15 minutes

Cooking time: 30 minutes

Servings: 8

Ingredients:

- 1 tablespoon curry paste
- 1 teaspoon curry

- 1 cup cream
- 1 pound salmon fillet
- ¼ cup garlic clove
- ½ tablespoon salt
- 1 teaspoon cilantro
- 1 teaspoon olive oil
- ¼ cup of fish sauce
- 1 onion
- 1 teaspoon red chili flakes
- 1 tablespoon fresh ginger
- 10 ounces keto dough

Directions:

1. Roll the keto dough using a rolling pin.

2. Spray the pressure cooker with the olive oil. Place the rolled dough into the pressure cooker.

3. Combine the curry paste, curry, cream, salt, cilantro, fish sauce, water, chili flakes, and fresh ginger in a mixing bowl and blend well and stir well.

4. Chop the salmon fillet and put it in the mixing bowl.

5. Add curry paste mixture and mix well. Put the fish mixture in the middle of the pie crust.

6. Grate the fresh ginger and sprinkle the top of the pie.

7. Peel the onion, slice it, and add it to the top of the fish pie and close the lid. Set the pressure cooker to "Pressure" mode.

8. Cook the dish on for 30 minutes. When the pie is cooked, remove it from the pressure cooker and slice it. Serve the pie warm.

Nutrition: calories 256, fat 8.5, fiber 5.3, carbs 13, protein 32.8

Mackerel Patties

Prep time: 10 minutes

Cooking time: 15 minutes

Servings: 6

Ingredients:

- 10 ounces mackerel
- 1 medium zucchini
- ½ cup coconut flour
- 2 eggs
- 1 teaspoon baking soda
- 1 tablespoon lemon juice
- 1 teaspoon oregano
- 1 tablespoon olive oil
- 2 garlic cloves
- 1 teaspoon red chili flakes

Directions:

1. Minced the mackerel and place it in a mixing bowl.

2. Wash the zucchini carefully and grate it.

3. Add the grated zucchini in the minced fish. Sprinkle the mixture with the baking soda, lemon juice, oregano, and chile flakes.

4. Peel the garlic cloves and slice them.

5. Add the garlic to the fish mixture. Whisk the eggs in the separate bowl.

6. Add the whisked eggs to the fish mixture.

7. Sprinkle the mixture with the coconut flour and knead the dough until smooth. Spray the pressure cooker with the olive oil.

8. Set the pressure cooker to "Sauté" mode.

9. Make medium-sized patties and put them into the pressure cooker. Sauté the dish for 5 minutes.

10. Flip the patties to cook on the other side. Sauté the dish for 10 minutes.

11. When the cooking time ends, open the pressure cooker lid and remove the cooked patties.

12. Let the dish rest. Let the dish rest briefly and serve.

Nutrition: calories 213, fat 13.7, fiber 3.8, carbs 7.1, protein 15

Oregano Whitebait

Prep time: 10 minutes

Cooking time: 10 minutes

Servings: 3

Ingredients:

- 1 teaspoon red chile flakes
- 1 tablespoon sour cream
- 4 tablespoons garlic sauce
- 1 pound whitebait
- 3 tablespoons butter
- ½ teaspoon sage
- 1 teaspoon oregano
- 1 teaspoon olive oil
- ½ cup almond flour
- ¼ cup milk
- 1 egg
- ½ teaspoon ground ginger

Directions:

1. Make fillets from the whitebait.

2. Combine the chile flakes, sage, oregano, and ground ginger in a bowl and mix well and stir.

3. Rub the whitebait fillets with the spice mixture.

4. Let the fish rest for 5 minutes.

5. Meanwhile, beat the egg in a separate bowl and whisk it. Add the milk and flour and stir until smooth.

6. Add the sour cream and stir.

7. Dip the whitebait fillets in the egg mixture. Set the pressure cooker to "Pressure" mode.

8. Add the butter into the pressure cooker and melt it.

9. Add the whitebait fillets and close the pressure cooker.

10. Cook the dish on for 10 minutes. When the cooking time ends, release the remaining pressure and open the pressure cooker lid.

11. Transfer the whitebait in a serving plate.

Nutrition: calories 472, fat 29.8, fiber 3.1, carbs 7.4, protein 43.2

Rosemary Mackerel Salad

Prep time: 10 minutes

Cooking time: 10 minutes

Servings: 6

Ingredients:

- 1 cup lettuce
- 8 ounces mackerel
- 1 teaspoon salt
- 1 teaspoon paprika
- 1 tablespoon olive oil
- ½ teaspoon rosemary
- 1 garlic clove
- ½ cup fish stock
- 1 teaspoon oregano
- 7 ounces tomatoes
- 1 large cucumber
- 1 red onion

Directions:

1. Wash the lettuce and chop it. Rub the mackerel with the salt, paprika, and rosemary.

2. Set the pressure cooker to "Pressure" mode.

3. Place the spiced mackerel into the pressure cooker. Add the fish stock and close the lid. Cook the dish on for 10 minutes.

4. Peel the garlic clove and slice it. Peel the red onion and slice it.

5. Combine the sliced onion with the chopped lettuce. Slice the cucumber and chop tomatoes.

6. Add the vegetables to the lettuce mixture. When the mackerel is cooked, remove it from the pressure cooker and let it rest briefly.

7. Chop the fish roughly. Add the chopped fish in the lettuce mixture.

8. Sprinkle the salad with the olive oil and stir it carefully using a so as not to damage the fish. Serve immediately.

Nutrition: calories 123, fat 6.5, fiber 1, carbs 5.29, protein 11

Monkfish Wine Stew

Prep time: 10 minutes

Cooking time: 30 minutes

Servings: 7

Ingredients:

- 1 pound monkfish fillet
- ½ cup white wine
- 1 teaspoon salt
- 1 teaspoon white pepper
- 1 medium carrot
- 2 white onions
- 1 cup fish stock
- 3 tablespoons fish sauce
- 1 tablespoon olive oil
- 1 teaspoon oregano
- ½ teaspoon fresh rosemary
- 1 cup of water
- 1 teaspoon sugar

- 1 teaspoon thyme
- 1 teaspoon coriander

Directions:

1. Chop the monkfish fillet roughly and sprinkle it with the salt, white pepper, fish sauce, oregano, fresh oregano, sugar, thyme, and coriander and stir well.

2. Let the fish rest for 5 minutes. Peel the onions and carrot and chop the vegetables. Set the pressure cooker to "Sauté" mode.

3. Put the chopped vegetables and monkfish into the pressure cooker. Sprinkle the mixture with the white wine, water, and olive oil.

4. Mix well and close the pressure cooker lid.

5. Cook the dish on for 30 minutes.

6. When the stew is cooked, open the pressure cooker lid and let the stew rest for 10 minutes. Transfer the stew to a serving bowl and serve.

Nutrition: calories 251, fat 14, fiber 5, carbs 15, protein 17

Eggplant Cod Chowder

Prep time: 10 minutes

Cooking time: 35 minutes

Servings: 8

Ingredients:

- 2 tablespoons fresh marjoram
- 1 teaspoon salt
- 3 cups of water
- 1 cup cream
- 1 onion
- 7 ounces eggplant
- 1 carrot
- 7 ounces cod
- 1 teaspoon ground black pepper
- 1 teaspoon butter
- 3 tablespoons chives
- ½ teaspoon nutmeg
- ½ cup dill

- 2 ounces fresh ginger

Directions:

1. Combine the water, cream, butter, and ground black pepper in a bowl and mix well and stir. Pour the cream mixture into the pressure cooker.

2. Sprinkle the mixture with the salt, chives, nutmeg, and fresh ginger.

3. Peel the onion, eggplants, and carrot.

4. Grate the carrot and put it into the pressure cooker. Dice the onion and chop the eggplant.

5. Set the pressure cooker to "Sauté" mode.

6. Add the cod and the vegetables to the pressure cooker. Sprinkle the mixture with the fresh marjoram.

7. Chop the dill.

8. Close the pressure cooker lid and cook the dish on for 35 minutes.

9. When the cooking time ends, release the remaining pressure and open the pressure cooker lid.

10. Ladle the chowder into serving bowls and sprinkle the bowls with the chopped dill. Serve the chowder hot.

Nutrition: calories 99, fat 3.1, fiber 3, carbs 11.7, protein 7.7

Salmon Mustard Tacos

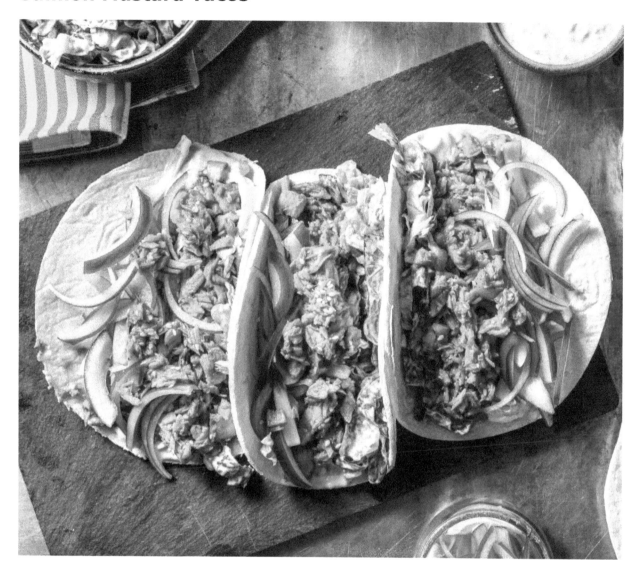

Prep time: 10 minutes

Cooking time: 10 minutes

Servings: 7

Ingredients:

- 7 almond tortilla
- 8 ounces salmon
- 2 red onions
- 2 red bell peppers
- 1 tablespoon mustard
- 1 tablespoon mayo sauce
- 1 garlic clove
- 2 tablespoons olive oil
- 1 teaspoon sesame seeds
- 1 teaspoon salt
- ¼ cup lettuce

Directions:

1. Combine mustard with the mayo sauce in a bowl and stir well. Sprinkle the salmon with the mustard sauce and coat the fish well.

2. Set the pressure cooker to "Steam" mode.

3. Spray the pressure cooker with the olive oil.

4. Add the salmon into the pressure cooker and close the lid. Cook the fish for 10 minutes.

5. Meanwhile, remove the seeds from the bell peppers.

6. Cut the bell peppers into strips. Peel the onion and slice it. Tear the lettuce.

7. Peel the garlic and mince the cloves. Sprinkle the tortilla shell with the minced garlic, salt, sesame seeds, and olive oil.

8. Add the bell pepper strips, sliced onions, and lettuce to the tortilla.

9. When the salmon is cooked, remove it from the pressure cooker.

10. Shred the salmon and put it in the tortilla and wrap the tacos.

Nutrition: calories 160, fat 9.8, fiber 2.5, carbs 8.7, protein 10.6

Sriracha Shrimp

Prep time: 10 minutes

Cooking time: 8 minutes

Servings: 6

Ingredients:

- 1 pound shrimp
- 3 tablespoons minced garlic
- 1 tablespoon sriracha
- 1 tablespoon sesame oil
- 1 teaspoon salt
- 1 teaspoon ground black pepper
- 1 teaspoon ground ginger
- ⅓ cup fish stock
- 1 tablespoon butter

Directions:

1. Peel the shrimp and combine them with the sriracha in a mixing bowl and stir well and sprinkle it with the sesame oil, minced garlic, salt, ground black pepper, ground ginger, and fish stock and stir well.

2. Toss everything well.

3. Place the sriracha shrimp into the pressure cooker. Set the pressure cooker to "Pressure" mode.

4. Add the butter and close the pressure cooker lid.

5. Cook the dish on for 8 minutes.

6. When the dish is cooked, remove the food from the pressure cooker. Let the dish rest. Let the dish rest briefly and serve.

Nutrition: calories 125, fat 5.4, fiber 0, carbs 2.33, protein 16

Tuna Noodles Salad

Prep time: 10 minutes

Cooking time: 12 minutes

Servings: 6

Ingredients:

- 5 ounces Shirataki noodles
- 1 pound tuna
- 1 tablespoon olive oil
- 1 teaspoon ground black pepper
- 3 tablespoons sour cream
- 1 teaspoon ground ginger
- 5 tablespoon fish stock
- 1 tablespoon soy sauce
- 6 ounces Parmesan cheese
- 1 cup black olives
- 1 cup hot water

Directions:

1. Combine the ground black pepper and ground ginger together in a bowl and mix well and stir.

2. Chop the tuna and add it to the ground black pepper mixture, stirring well. Cut the cheese into the cubes. Set the pressure cooker to "Steam" mode.

3. Place the chopped tuna into the pressure cooker and cook it for 12 minutes.

4. Combine the sliced black olives, cheese cubes, olive oil in the mixing bowl. Add soy sauce and fish stock.

5. Sprinkle the mixture with the sour cream. When the tuna is cooked, release the pressure and open the instant lid.

6. Chill the chopped tuna. Combine hot water and noodles together and let them sit for 15 minutes.

7. Rinse the noodles and place them in the black olive mixture. Add the chilled chopped tuna and toss the salad gently. Transfer the salad to serving bowls.

Nutrition: calories 301, fat 18.3, fiber 3.4, carbs 3.3, protein 30.2

Oregano Snapper

Prep time: 10 minutes

Cooking time: 15 minutes

Servings: 4

Ingredients:

- ½ cup tomato juice
- 1 large onion
- ½ teaspoon salt
- 1 tablespoon basil
- 1 teaspoon oregano
- 4 garlic cloves
- 1 tablespoon butter
- ½ cup chicken stock
- 1 pound snapper
- 2 tablespoons fish sauce

Directions:

1. Remove the skin from the snapper, make small slits into the surface of the skin, and set aside.

2. Peel the onion and slice it. Combine the salt, basil, oregano, and fish sauce together in a mixing bowl and stir well.

3. Rub the peeled fish with the spice mixture. Peel the garlic cloves and slice them. Set the pressure cooker to "Pressure" mode.

4. Fill the snapper with the sliced garlic and onion and place the fish into the pressure cooker.

5. Add tomato juice and close the lid.

6. Cook the dish on mode for 15 minutes.

7. When the cooking time ends, remove the snapper from the pressure cooker carefully so as not to damage the fish.

8. Sprinkle the fish with the tomato juice from the pressure cooker. Let it rest briefly and serve.

Nutrition: calories 204, fat 5.1, fiber 1.2, carbs 6.5, protein 31.2

Garlic Mussel Soup

Prep time: 10 minutes

Cooking time: 8 minutes

Servings: 6

Ingredients:

- 1 cup cream
- 3 cups chicken stock
- 2 tablespoons olive oil
- 8 ounces mussels
- 1 tablespoon minced garlic
- ½ chili paper
- 1 teaspoon red chile flakes
- 1 onion
- ½ tablespoon salt
- ½ cup parsley
- 7 ounces shallot
- 1 tablespoon lime juice
- 1 teaspoon black-eyed peas

Directions:

1. Peel the onion and slice it. Chop the shallot and parsley.

2. Set the pressure cooker to "Sauté" mode. Pour the olive oil into the pressure cooker. Add the shallot.

3. Add onion into the pressure cooker and cook the dish on a dish for 4 minutes, stirring frequently.

4. Add chicken stock, cream, minced garlic, chili flakes, salt, lime juice, and black-eyed peas.

5. Add mussels and sprinkle the mixture with the chopped parsley. Close the pressure cooker lid.

6. Set the pressure cooker to "Pressure" mode. Cook the dish for 4 minutes.

7. When the cooking time ends, release the pressure and open the pressure cooker lid. Ladle the mussel soup into serving bowls.

Nutrition: calories 231, fat 14.7, fiber 1, carbs 15.63, protein 10

Doughy Salmon Bars

Prep time: 15 minutes

Cooking time: 25 minutes

Servings: 6

Ingredients:

- 9 ounces keto dough
- 1 tablespoon olive oil
- 1 teaspoon butter
- ½ teaspoon rosemary
- 1 teaspoon salt
- 9 ounces smoked salmon
- 6 ounces mozzarella cheese
- 1 teaspoon fresh thyme
- 1 tablespoon tomato paste
- 1 teaspoon garlic sauce

Directions:

1. Roll the dough using a rolling pin.

2. Spread the pressure cooker vessel with the butter. Place the rolled dough into the pressure cooker.

3. Sprinkle the dough with the olive oil and rosemary.

4. Chop the smoked salmon and sprinkle it with the salt and mix well and stir. Slice the mozzarella cheese.

5. Sprinkle the keto dough with the garlic sauce and tomato paste. Add the smoked salmon and sliced cheese.

6. Sprinkle the dish with the fresh thyme and close the lid. Cook the dish on the "Sauté" mode for 25 minutes.

7. When the cooking time ends, open the pressure cooker and let the dish rest. Cut the dish into the squares and serve.

Nutrition: calories 310, fat 11.7, fiber 5.9, carbs 11.1, protein 40.5

Halibut with Ginger Sauce

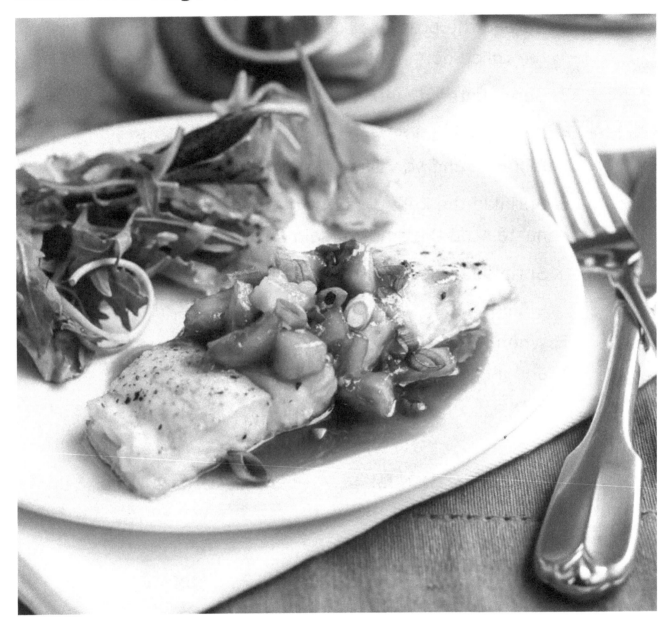

Prep time: 10 minutes

Cooking time: 9 minutes

Servings: 6

Ingredients:

- 1 pound halibut
- 1 tablespoon butter
- 3 tablespoons fish sauce
- 1 teaspoon rosemary
- 1 tablespoon cream
- 1 teaspoon ground white pepper
- ½ cup of soy sauce
- 2 tablespoons fresh ginger
- 1 teaspoon olive oil
- 1 teaspoon ground ginger

Directions:

1. Cut the halibut into the fillets and.

2. Sprinkle the halibut with the rosemary and ground white pepper. Set the pressure cooker to "Sauté" mode.

3. Add the butter into the pressure cooker and melt it at the sauté mode. Place the fish into the pressure cooker.

4. Sauté the halibut fillets into the pressure cooker for 2 minutes on both sides.

5. Combine the fish sauce, cream, soy sauce, fresh ginger, olive oil, and ground ginger together in the bowl and mix well.

6. Sprinkle the halibut fillet with the ginger sauce and close the pressure cooker lid. Cook the dish on "Pressure" mode for 5 minutes.

7. When the cooking time ends, open the pressure cooker lid and remove the halibut fillets from the pressure cooker vessel gently so not to damage the dish and let it rest before serving.

Nutrition: calories 240, fat 17.5, fiber 1, carbs 7.01, protein 13

Snapper with Onions

Prep time: 10 minutes

Cooking time: 20 minutes

Servings: 4

Ingredients:

- 1 pound snapper
- 2 white onions
- ½ cup dill
- 1 tablespoon olive oil
- 3 garlic cloves
- 1 teaspoon Erythritol
- ½ tablespoon of sea salt
- 1 teaspoon turmeric
- 1 teaspoon oregano
- ½ teaspoon cumin
- 1 teaspoon ground coriander
- 1 teaspoon dried celery root
- 4 ounces mushrooms

Directions:

1. Peel the snapper and cut it crosswise. Sprinkle the fish with sea salt. Peel the onions and dice them.

2. Peel the garlic cloves and slice them.

3. Pour the olive oil into the pressure cooker and preheat it on the "Sauté" mode. Add the diced onions and sliced garlic.

4. Stir the mixture and cook it for 4 minutes and mix well. Remove the cooked onion mixture from the pressure cooker and chill it well.

5. Chop the dill and sprinkle the cooked onion mixture with it. Add Erythritol, turmeric, oregano, cumin, ground coriander, and celery root.

6. Dice the mushrooms.

7. Add the mushrooms to the onion mixture. Fill the snapper with the onion mixture and wrap the fish in aluminum foil.

8. Place the wrapped fish on the trivet and put it into the pressure cooker. Cook the dish on the "Steam" mode for 20 minutes.

9. When the dish is cooked, open the pressure cooker lid and remove the fish. Discard the aluminum foil and chop the fish, if desired, before serving.

Nutrition: calories 230, fat 6.1, fiber 2.7, carbs 12, protein 32.7

Coconut Cod

Prep time: 10 minutes

Cooking time: 10 minutes

Servings: 5

Ingredients:

- 12 ounces cod fillet
- 3 eggs
- 1 cup coconut flour
- ⅓ cup pork rinds
- 1 teaspoon salt
- 2 tablespoons olive oil
- 1 teaspoon ground white pepper
- 1 teaspoon ground ginger
- 1 tablespoon turmeric
- 2 teaspoons sesame seeds
- ¼ teaspoon red chili flakes

Directions:

1. Whisk the eggs in a mixing bowl using a hand mixer. Add the coconut flour and continue to mix the mixture until smooth.

2. Sprinkle the cod fillets with the salt, ground ginger, ground white pepper, and chili flakes. Add turmeric and mix well.

3. Dip the cod fillets in the egg mixture.

4. Sprinkle the fish with the pork rinds and sesame seeds.

5. Pour olive oil into the pressure cooker and preheat it on the "Sauté" mode. Add the cod fillets and cook them for 5 minutes on each side.

6. When the cod fillets are cooked, remove them from the pressure cooker and transfer the dish to paper towel drain.

7. Rest briefly before serving.

Nutrition: calories 198, fat 12, fiber 1.6, carbs 3.5, protein 19.9

Sweet Creamy Mackerel

Prep time: 10 minutes

Cooking time: 28 minutes

Servings: 5

Ingredients:

- 1 teaspoon Erythritol
- 2 tablespoons water
- ¼ cup cream
- 1 pound mackerel
- 1 teaspoon ground white pepper
- 3 tablespoons oregano
- 1 teaspoon olive oil
- ¼ cup of water
- ¼ teaspoon cinnamon

Directions:

1. Chop the mackerel roughly and sprinkle it with the water, Erythritol, ground white pepper, olive oil, and cinnamon and stir well.

2. Place the fish mixture into the pressure cooker. Add water and close the lid. Cook the dish on "Sauté" mode for 20 minutes.

3. Do not stir the dish during the cooking.

4. When the cooking time ends, remove the dish from the pressure cooker.

5. Transfer to serving plates and serve.

Nutrition: calories 263, fat 18.1, fiber 1.3, carbs 3.3, protein 22.1

Chili Anchovy

Prep time: 15 minutes

Cooking time: 8 minutes

Servings: 3

Ingredients:

- 1 red chile pepper
- 10 ounces anchovies
- 4 tablespoons butter
- 1 teaspoon of sea salt
- ½ teaspoon paprika
- 1 teaspoon red chile flakes
- 1 tablespoon basil
- 1 teaspoon dried dill
- 1 teaspoon rosemary
- ⅓ cup breadcrumbs

Directions:

1. Remove the seeds from the chile pepper and slice it.

2. Combine the chile flakes, paprika, sea salt, basil, dry dill, and rosemary together in a shallow bowl and stir well.

3. Sprinkle the anchovies with the spice mixture. Combine well using your hands.

4. Add sliced chile pepper and Let the mixture rest for 10 minutes.

5. Set the pressure cooker to "Sauté" mode. Add the butter into the pressure cooker and melt it.

6. Dip the spiced anchovies in the breadcrumbs and put the fish in the melted butter.

7. Cook the anchovies for 4 minutes on each side. When the fish is cooked, remove it from the pressure cooker and drain it on a paper towel to remove any excess oil.

8. Serve immediately.

Nutrition: calories 356, fat 25, fiber 1, carbs 4.17, protein 28

Marinated Shrimps

Prep time: 20 minutes

Cooking time: 7 minutes

Servings: 3

Ingredients:

- 2 tablespoons fresh cilantro
- 2 tablespoons apple cider vinegar
- 1 tablespoon lemon juice
- ½ teaspoon lemon zest
- ½ tablespoon salt
- ¼ cup white wine
- 1 teaspoon brown sugar
- ½ teaspoon ground ginger
- 1 tablespoon olive oil
- ½ tablespoon minced garlic
- 1 teaspoon nutmeg
- 1 cup of water
- .5½ pound shrimp

- 1 cup parsley

Directions:

1. Chop the cilantro and parsley.

2. Combine the lemon juice, apple cider vinegar, lemon zest, salt, white wine, and sugar together in a mixing bowl.

3. Stir the mixture until sugar and salt are dissolved. Peel the shrimp and devein and put them in the lemon juice mixture.

4. Add the chopped cilantro and parsley and stir well. Add ground ginger, olive oil, nutmeg, and water.

5. Mix up the shrimp mixture well and let it marinate for 15 minutes. Set the pressure cooker to "Pressure" mode.

6. Transfer the marinated shrimp into the pressure cooker and cook the dish for 7 minutes.

7. When the cooking time ends, release the remaining pressure and open the pressure cooker lid.

8. Serve the shrimp warm or keep them in the marinated liquid in your refrigerator.

Nutrition: calories 143, fat 6, fiber 1, carbs 5.63, protein 16

Shrimp Lemon Cocktail

Prep time: 10 minutes

Cooking time: 1 minute

Servings: 6

Ingredients:

- 16 oz shrimps, peeled
- 1 cup low carb ketchup
- ½ tablespoon lemon juice
- 1 teaspoon horseradish, grated
- ¼ teaspoon white pepper
- ½ teaspoon salt
- 1 cup water, for cooking

Directions:

1. Pour water and insert the steamer rack in the instant pot.

2. Sprinkle the shrimps with salt and place in the steamer rack.

3. Cook the seafood for 0 minutes on manual mode (high pressure). Make a quick pressure release and transfer the shrimps in the serving plate.

4.   Then make shrimp cocktail sauce: in the sauce bowl, mix up together low carb ketchup, lemon juice, horseradish, and white pepper.

5.   Dip the shrimps in the sauce.

Nutrition value/serving: calories 99, fat 1.3, fiber 0.1, carbs 1.3, protein 17.3

Cheddar Mussels Casserole

Prep time: 10 minutes

Cooking time: 13 minutes

Servings: 4

Ingredients:

- 9 oz mussels, canned
- 1 cup cauliflower, chopped
- ½ cup Cheddar cheese, shredded
- ½ cup heavy cream
- 1 teaspoon Italian seasonings
- 1 teaspoon olive oil
- 1 teaspoon salt
- 1 tablespoon fresh dill, chopped
- 1 cup water, for cooking

Directions:

1. Pour water and insert the trivet in the instant pot.

2. Place the cauliflower on the trivet and cook it on manual mode (high pressure) for 3 minutes. Then make a quick pressure release.

3. Transfer the cauliflower in the instant pot casserole mold.

4. Add canned mussels, cheese, heavy cream, Italian seasonings, olive oil, salt, and dill.

5. Mix up the casserole and cover it with foil.

6. Place the casserole mold on the trivet and close the lid.

7. Cook the casserole for 10 minutes on manual mode (high pressure).

8. When the time is over, make a quick pressure release.

9. Mix up the casserole with the help of the spoon before serving.

Nutrition value/serving: calories 185, fat 13.2, fiber 0.7, carbs 4.9, protein 12.1

Ricotta Shrimps

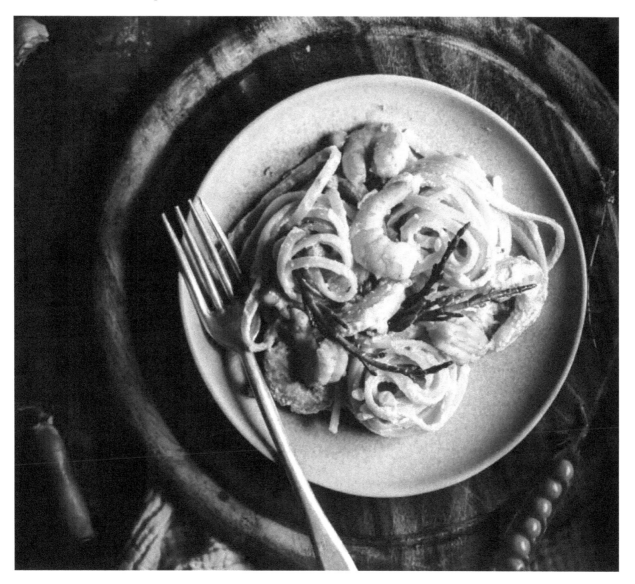

Prep time: 10 minutes

Cooking time: 1 minute

Servings:4

Ingredients:

- 11 oz shrimps, peeled

- ½ cup of coconut milk

- 1 tablespoon ricotta cheese

- 2 tablespoons fresh parsley, chopped

- 1 teaspoon lime juice

- ¼ teaspoon chili powder

- ¼ teaspoon ground black pepper

- 1 red onion, chopped

- 1 cup water, for cooking

Directions:

1. Pour water and insert the steamer rack in the instant pot.

2. Put the shrimps in the rack and close the lid.

3. Cook them on manual mode (high pressure) for 1 minute. When the time is over, make a quick pressure release and transfer the shrimps in the salad bowl.

4. In the separated bowl mix up together coconut milk, ricotta cheese, fresh parsley, lime juice, chili powder, and ground black pepper. The sauce is cooked.

5. Combine together shrimps with chopped red onion.

6. Add sauce and mix it up.

Nutrition value/serving: calories 180, fat 8.9, fiber 1.4, carbs 6, protein 19.3

Butter Scallops

Prep time: 10 minutes

Cooking time: 7 minutes

Servings: 4

Ingredients:

- 1-pound scallops
- 3 tablespoons butter
- ½ teaspoon dried rosemary
- ¼ teaspoon salt

Directions:

1. Put butter in the instant pot.

2. Set sauté mode and melt butter (it will take approximately 3 minutes.

3. Add dried rosemary and salt. Stir the butter.

4. Then place the scallops in the hot butter in one layer.

5. Cook them on sauté mode for 2 minutes.

6. Then flip the scallops on another side and cook for 2 minutes more.

7. Serve the scallops with hot butter.

Nutrition value/serving: calories 177, fat 9.5, fiber 0.1, carbs 2.8, protein 19.1

Cajun Crab Casserole

Prep time: 10 minutes

Cooking time: 15 minutes

Servings: 6

Ingredients:

- ½ cup celery stalks, chopped
- ½ white onion, diced
- 3 eggs, beaten
- 1 tablespoon dried parsley
- 10 oz crab meat, chopped, canned
- 1 teaspoon Cajun seasonings
- ½ cup white Cheddar cheese, shredded
- ½ teaspoon salt
- ½ teaspoon ground black pepper
- ½ teaspoon cayenne pepper
- ½ cup heavy cream
- 1 teaspoon sesame oil

Directions:

1.   Heat up the instant pot on sauté mode for 3 minutes and add sesame oil.

2.   Add diced onion and cook it for 2 minutes. Stir it well.

3.   Switch off the instant pot.

4.   Add celery stalk in the onion and mix up.

5.   Then add beaten eggs, dried parsley, crab meat, Cajun seasonings, cheese, salt, ground black pepper, cayenne pepper, and heavy cream.

6.   Stir the casserole carefully with the help of a spatula and close the lid.

7.   Cook the meal on stew mode for 10 minutes.

Nutrition value/serving: calories 159, fat 9.7, fiber 0.4, carbs 2.8, protein 11.5

Crab Melt with Monterey Jack

Prep time: 15 minutes

Cooking time: 8 minutes

Servings: 4

Ingredients:

- 1 large zucchini
- 1 teaspoon avocado oil
- ½ cup Monterey Jack cheese, shredded
- 1 green bell pepper, finely chopped
- 9 oz crab meat, chopped
- 2 tablespoons ricotta cheese
- 1 cup water, for cooking

Directions:

1. Trim the ends of zucchini and slice it lengthwise into 4 slices.

2. Then pour water in the instant pot and insert the trivet.

3. Place the zucchini slices in the baking mold.

4. Brush them with avocado oil gently.

5.   After this, in the mixing bowl combine together Monterey Jack cheese, bell pepper, crab meat, and ricotta cheese.

6.   Spread the mixture over the zucchini and transfer it on the trivet.

7.   Close the instant pot lid and cook the meal on manual mode (high pressure) for 8 minutes.

8.   When the time is over, make a quick pressure release.

Nutrition value/serving: calories 144, fat 6.4, fiber 1.3, carbs 6.7, protein 13.6

Lemongrass Baked Snapper

Prep time: 10 minutes

Cooking time: 10 minutes

Servings: 4

Ingredients:

- 1-pound snapper, trimmed, cleaned
- 1 tablespoon lemongrass
- 1 tablespoon sage
- 1 teaspoon avocado oil
- 1 teaspoon salt
- 1 teaspoon red pepper
- 1 cup water, for cooking

Directions:

1. Pour water and insert trivet in the instant pot.

2. Rub the fish with salt and red pepper.

3. Then fill it with sage and lemongrass.

4. Brush the fish with avocado oil and transfer on the trivet.

5. Close the lid and cook the snapper for 10 minutes on manual mode (high pressure).

6.   When the time is over, make a quick pressure release and open the lid.

7.   Remove the sage and lemongrass from the fish.

Nutrition value/serving: calories 151, fat 2.2, fiber 0.7, carbs 2.9, protein 27.9

Salmon Onion Salad

Prep time: 10 minutes

Cooking time: 8 minutes

Servings: 2

Ingredients:

- ½ cup curly kale, chopped
- 7 oz salmon fillet, chopped
- 1 teaspoon onion flakes
- ½ teaspoon salt
- 1 teaspoon coconut oil
- 1 teaspoon olive oil
- ½ teaspoon chili flakes
- ¼ cup cherry tomatoes, halved

Directions:

1. Place coconut oil in the instant pot and heat it up on sauté mode.

2. When the coconut oil is melted, add salmon fillet.

3. Sprinkle the fish with salt and chili flakes. Cook it for 2 minutes from each side on sauté mode.

4.   Then transfer the cooked salmon in the salad bowl.

5.   Add curly kale, onion flakes, salt, olive oil, and halved cherry tomatoes.

6.   Shake the salad.

Nutrition value/serving: calories 202, fat 11.2, fiber 2.2, carbs 6, protein 21.7

Cod Loin

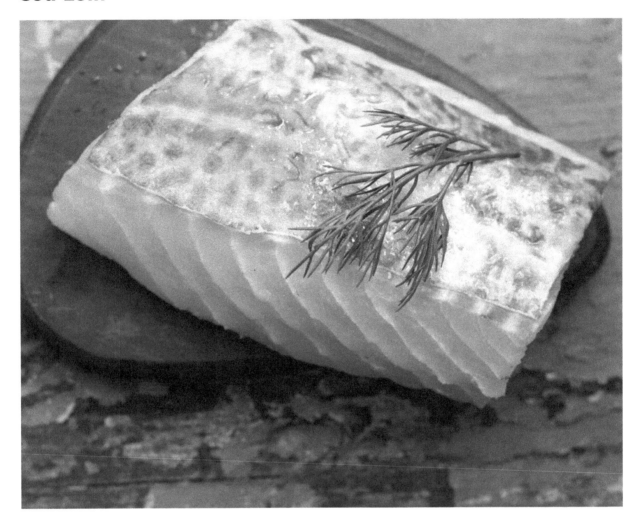

Prep time: 10 minutes

Cooking time: 15 minutes

Servings: 2

Ingredients:

- 8 oz cod loin
- 1 tablespoon oregano
- ¼ teaspoon chili flakes

- 3 tablespoons butter

- ½ teaspoon salt

- ¼ teaspoon minced ginger

Directions:

1. Put butter and chili flakes in the instant pot bowl.

2. Set sauté mode and melt the mixture.

3. Add minced ginger, salt, oregano, and stir it.

4. Then arrange the cod loin inside.

5. Cook it on sauté mode for 6 minutes from each side.

6. Serve the fish topped with hot butter mixture from the instant pot.

Nutrition value/serving: calories 251, fat 18.5, fiber 1, carbs 1.6, protein 20.5

Salmon in Cream Sauce

Prep time: 5 minutes

Cooking time: 15 minutes

Servings: 4

Ingredients:

- 16 oz salmon fillet
- 1 cup heavy cream
- 1 teaspoon minced garlic
- 1 tablespoon fresh parsley, chopped
- 1 teaspoon chives, chopped
- 1 oz Parmesan, grated
- 1 cup water, for cooking

Directions:

1. Mix up together water and minced garlic and pour the liquid in the instant pot. Insert trivet and place a salmon fillet in it.

2. Close the lid and cook the fish on steam mode for 5 minutes. Then allow the natural pressure release for 5 minutes and transfer the fish on the plate. Cut it into servings.

3. After this, remove the liquid from the instant pot. Discard the trivet.

4. Pour heavy cream in the instant pot.

5. Add parsley and chives.

6. Bring the liquid to boil on sauté mode.

7. Then add cheese and switch off the instant pot.

8. Stir the liquid carefully until the cheese is melted.

9. Pour the cooked cream sauce over the salmon.

Nutrition value/serving: calories 278, fat 19.6, fiber 0.1, carbs 1.4, protein 25

Kohlrabi Gratin with Salmon

Prep time: 10 minutes

Cooking time: 14 minutes

Servings: 3

Ingredients:

- 8 oz salmon fillet, chopped
- ¼ teaspoon ground black pepper
- ½ teaspoon salt
- 4 oz kohlrabi, chopped
- ½ cup heavy cream
- 1 tablespoon almond meal
- 1 teaspoon lemon juice
- 1 teaspoon sesame oil
- 3 oz Provolone cheese, grated
- 1 cup water, for cooking

Directions:

1. Pour water and insert the steamer rack in the instant pot.

2. Place kohlrabi in the steamer and cook it on steam mode for 4 minutes.

3. Then make a quick pressure release.

4. Brush the instant pot pan mold with sesame oil.

5. Place the salmon in it.

6. Then sprinkle the fish with salt and ground black pepper.

7. Top the fish with kohlrabi.

8. After this, sprinkle the mixture with lemon juice, almond meal, heavy cream, and Provolone cheese.

9. Place the mold in the steamer rack and close the lid.

10. Cook the gratin on manual mode (high pressure) for 10 minutes.

11. Then make quick pressure realize.

Nutrition value/serving: calories 304, fat 22.2, fiber 1.7, carbs 4.1, protein 23.4

Zucchini Mussel Chowder

Prep time: 10 minutes

Cooking time: 30 minutes

Servings: 4

Ingredients:

- 1 cup heavy cream
- 1 cup chicken broth
- 6 oz mussels, canned
- 1 zucchini, chopped
- 1 teaspoon paprika
- ½ teaspoon salt
- 1 onion, diced
- 1 teaspoon coconut oil

Directions:

1. Toss coconut oil in the instant pot.

2. Add onion and cook the ingredients on sauté mode for 5 minutes.

3. Then stir well and cook for 3 minutes more.

4. After this, add zucchini and salt.

5.   Saute the ingredients for 2 minutes more.

6.   Add paprika, salt, chicken stock, and heavy cream.

7.   Close the lid and cook the chowder on soup mode for 20 minutes.

8.   Then open the lid and with the help of the immersion blender, blend the chowder until it gets the creamy texture.

9.   Add mussels and cook the chowder for 5 minutes more on sauté mode.

Nutrition value/serving: calories 180, fat 13.7, fiber 1.3, carbs 7.2, protein 7.9

Turmeric Salmon Skewers

Prep time: 15 minutes

Cooking time: 5 minutes

Servings: 4

Ingredients:

- 1-pound salmon fillet, fresh, cubed
- 1 tablespoon paprika
- ½ teaspoon salt
- ½ teaspoon ground turmeric
- 1 teaspoon avocado oil
- ½ teaspoon lemon juice
- 1 cup water, for cooking

Directions:

1. Make the sauce: mix up together paprika, salt, ground turmeric, avocado oil, and lemon juice.

2. Then coat the salmon cubes in the sauce well and string on the wooden skewers.

3. Pour water and insert trivet in the instant pot.

4. Arrange the salmon skewers on the trivet and close the lid.

5.   Cook the meal on manual mode (high pressure) for 5 minutes.

6.   Then make a quick pressure release and remove the fish from the instant pot.

Nutrition value/serving: calories 158, fat 7.4, fiber 0.8, carbs 1.2, protein 22.3

ProvoloneTuscan Shrimps

Prep time: 10 minutes

Cooking time: 25 minutes

Servings: 4

Ingredients:

- 1-pound shrimps, peeled
- ¼ teaspoon minced garlic
- 1 teaspoon butter
- 1 teaspoon coconut oil
- ½ white onion, diced
- 1 teaspoon apple cider vinegar
- 1 cup heavy cream
- ¼ teaspoon salt
- ½ teaspoon ground black pepper
- 2 cups spinach, chopped
- 3 oz Provolone cheese, grated
- 1 tablespoon almond flour
- 1 teaspoon Italian seasonings
- 1 teaspoon dried cilantro
- ¼ cup of water

Directions:

1.	Heat up instant pot on sauté mode for 3 minutes.

2.	Then place butter and coconut oil inside.

3.	Heat up the ingredients for 2 minutes and add minced garlic and diced onion.

4.	Add apple cider vinegar and stir the ingredients.

5.	Sauté them for 5 minutes. Stir the mixture from time to time.

6.	Then add salt, ground black pepper, cilantro, Italian seasonings, and stir well.

7.	Add water and bring the mixture to boil on sauté mode. Add spinach and almond flour.

8.	Stir it well and cook for 3 minutes.

9.	Then add heavy cream and shrimps.

10.	Cook the meal on sauté mode for 10 minutes.

Nutrition value/serving: calories 385, fat 24.7, fiber 1.4, carbs 6.7, protein 34

Garlic Parmesan Scallops

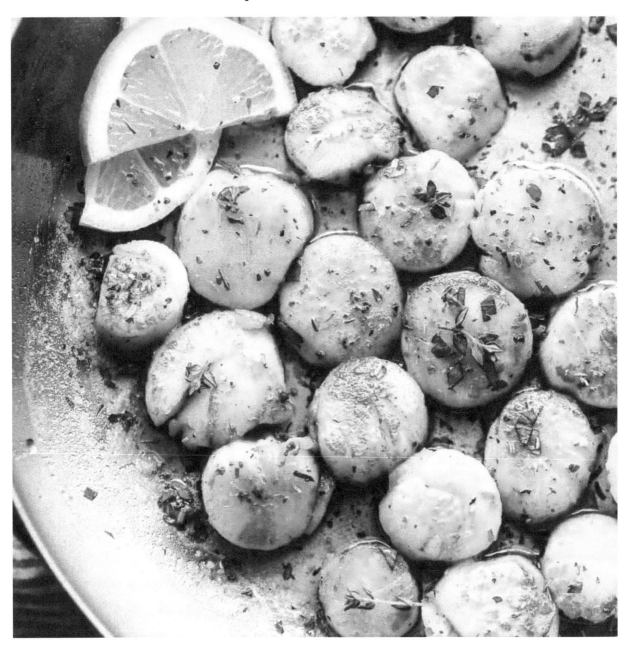

Prep time: 8 minutes

Cooking time: 11 minutes

Servings: 4

Ingredients:

- 11 oz scallops

- 4 oz Parmesan, grated

- 1 tablespoon butter, melted

- ½ teaspoon avocado oil

- 1 teaspoon garlic powder

Directions:

1. Brush scallops with butter and sprinkle with garlic powder.

2. Brush the instant pot bowl with avocado oil and heat it up for 3 minutes on sauté mode.

3. Then place the scallops in the instant pot in one layer and cook them for 3 minutes.

4. Flip the scallops and top with grated Parmesan.

5. Close the lid and sauté the meal for 5 minutes more.

Nutrition value/serving: calories 188, fat 6.9, fiber 0.1, carbs 3.4, protein 22.4

Seafood Bisque

Prep time: 5 minutes

Cooking time: 10 minutes

Servings: 3

Ingredients:

- 1 tablespoon coconut oil
- 1 oz leek, chopped
- ½ red onion, diced
- 1 teaspoon celery, chopped
- ½ teaspoon ground thyme
- ½ teaspoon lemon zest, grated
- 3 tablespoons cream cheese
- 1 cup chicken broth
- 1 tablespoon scallions, chopped
- 1 oz bacon, chopped, cooked
- ½ teaspoon salt
- 9 oz shrimps, peeled

Directions:

1. Put coconut oil in the instant pot and melt it on sauté mode for 2 minutes.

2. Then add leek, red onion, and celery.

3. Sprinkle the ingredients with ground thyme, lemon zest, and salt. Mix up well and cook on sauté mode for 4 minutes.

4. Then add cream cheese and stir well until homogenous.

5. Then and chicken stock and shrimps. Mix up the meal well and close the lid.

6. Cook it on manual mode (high pressure) for 2 minutes.

7. When the time is over, make a quick pressure release.

8. Top the cooked meal with bacon and scallions.

Nutrition value/serving: calories 253, fat 13.9, fiber 0.7, carbs 5.4, protein 25.7

Lobster Bisque

Prep time: 10 minutes

Cooking time: 15 minutes

Servings: 4

Ingredients:

- 1 teaspoon tomato paste
- 1 tablespoon celery, grated
- 1 white onion, diced
- ¼ teaspoon minced garlic
- 1 tablespoon butter
- 3 cups chicken broth
- 1 tablespoon ground paprika
- ½ teaspoon ground black pepper
- ½ cup heavy cream
- 4 lobster tails
- ½ teaspoon salt
- 1 tablespoon chives, chopped

Directions:

1. Melt the butter in the instant pot on sauté mode for 3 minutes.

2. Then add celery and onion. Cook the vegetables for 2 minutes.

3. After this, stir them well and add minced garlic. Mix up well.

4. Add lobster tails and cook them for 1 minute from each side.

5. After this, mix up together tomato paste and heavy cream.

6. Add the liquid in the instant pot.

7. Then add chicken broth, ground black pepper, ground paprika, and salt. Close the lid.

8. Cook the bisque for 3 minutes on manual mode (high pressure).

9. When the time is over, make a quick pressure release.

10. Top the meal with chopped chives.

Nutrition value/serving: calories 170, fat 9.7, fiber 1.4, carbs 5.2, protein 4.7

Lemon Lobster

Prep time: 10 minutes

Cooking time: 8 minutes

Servings: 3

Ingredients:

- 12 oz lobster tails
- 1 tablespoon tarragon
- 1 tablespoon lemon juice
- 2 tablespoons butter, melted
- ¼ teaspoon salt
- 1 cup water, for cooking

Directions:

1. With the help of the scissors and knife trim and clean the lobster tails from shells.

2. Then pour water and insert the steamer rack in the instant pot.

3. Arrange the lobster tails on the rack and close the lid.

4. Cook the seafood for 3 minutes on manual mode (high pressure).

5.   When the time is over, make a quick pressure release and open the lid.

6.   Transfer the lobsters on the plate and clean the instant pot.

7.   Remove the steamer rack from the instant pot.

8.   Put the melted butter, tarragon, lemon juice, and salt in the instant pot and cook it for 3 minutes on sauté mode.

9.   Top every lobster tail with fragrant butter liquid.

Nutrition value/serving: calories 172, fat 8.7, fiber 0.1, carbs 0.4, protein 21.8

Milky Mussels

Prep time: 10 minutes

Cooking time: 8 minutes

Servings: 5

Ingredients:

- 2 garlic cloves, diced

- 1 white onion, diced

- 1 tablespoon fresh parsley, chopped

- 1 cup chicken broth

- ¼ cup of coconut milk

- 1 tablespoon avocado oil

- 1 tablespoon lemon juice

- 1-pound fresh mussels

Directions:

1. Pour avocado oil in the instant pot.

2. Add diced garlic and onion.

3. Cook the vegetables on sauté mode for 4 minutes. Stir them after 2 minutes of cooking.

4. Then add parsley, lemon juice, and coconut milk.

5.   Mix up the mixture and cook it for 1 minute.

6.   Add mussels and chicken broth,

7.   Close the lid and cook the meal on manual mode (high pressure) for 3 minutes.

8.   When the time is over, make a quick pressure release.

Nutrition value/serving: calories 129, fat 5.6, fiber 0.9, carbs 6.9, protein 12.4

Tuna Egg Cakes

Prep time: 15 minutes

Cooking time: 4 minutes

Servings: 4

Ingredients:

- 10 oz tuna, canned
- 1 egg, beaten
- 1 teaspoon dried oregano
- ½ teaspoon salt
- 1 teaspoon ground coriander
- 3 tablespoons coconut flour
- ½ teaspoon chili flakes
- 1 cup water, for cooking

Directions:

1. Place the canned tuna in the bowl and smash it with the help of the fork.

2. When the tuna is smooth, add egg, dried oregano, salt, ground coriander, coconut flour, and chili flakes.

3. Stir the tuna cakes mixture well.

4.   After this, pour water and insert the steamer rack in the instant pot.

5.   With the help of the scooper make the medium size tuna cakes and place them on the trivet on one layer.

6.   Close the lid and cook the meal on manual mode (high pressure) for 5 minutes. Then allow the natural pressure release for 5 minutes more and transfer the tuna cakes on the plate.

Nutrition value/serving: calories 175, fat 7.8, fiber 2.4, carbs 3.7, protein 21.4

Salmon under Parmesan

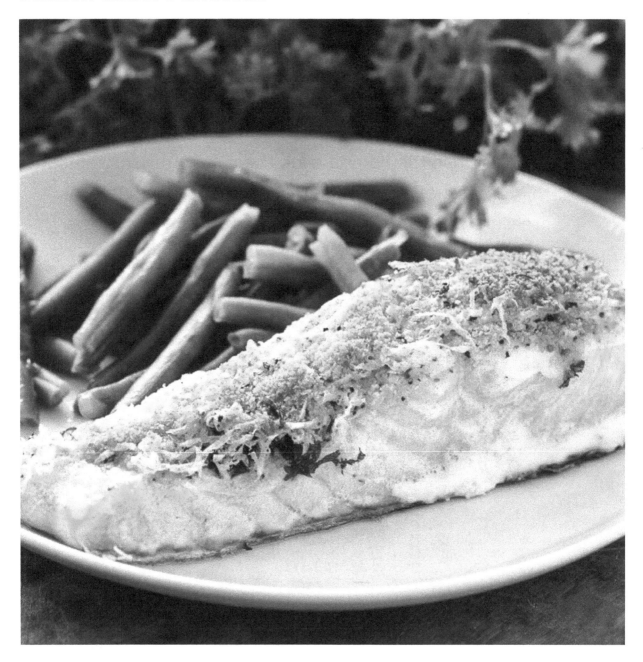

Prep time: 10 minutes

Cooking time: 11 minutes

Servings: 4

Ingredients:

- 1-pound salmon fillet
- 1 teaspoon chili flakes
- ¼ teaspoon cayenne pepper
- 1 teaspoon olive oil
- ½ teaspoon ground paprika
- ½ teaspoon dried thyme
- 4 oz Parmesan, grated
- 1 cup water, for cooking

Directions:

1. In the shallow bowl combine together chili flakes, cayenne pepper, ground paprika, and dried thyme.

2. Then rub the salmon fillet with spices.

3. After this, brush the fish fillet with olive oil.

4. Heat up the instant pot on sauté mode for 3 minutes.

5. Then place the salmon fillet in the hot instant pot and cook for 2 minutes from each side.

6. Then remove the fish from the instant pot.

7. Clean the instant pot and pour water inside.

8. Insert the steamer rack and line it with foil.

9. Place the salmon fillet in the instant pot and top with grated Parmesan.

10. Close the lid and cook the meal on manual (high pressure) for 5 minutes. Then make a quick pressure release.

11. Transfer the cooked fish on the plate and cut it into servings.

Nutrition value/serving: calories 253, fat 14.3, fiber 0.2, carbs 1.3, protein 31.2

Salmon Poppers

Prep time: 15 minutes

Cooking time: 10 minutes

Servings: 6

Ingredients:

- 10 oz salmon fillet, chopped
- 3 eggs, beaten
- 1 tablespoon pork rinds
- 1 jalapeno pepper, chopped
- 1 tablespoon cream cheese
- ¼ teaspoon garlic powder
- 1 teaspoon dried oregano
- ½ teaspoon salt
- 1 tablespoon coconut oil
- ½ teaspoon onion powder

Directions:

1. Put the salmon fillet in the food processor.

2. Add egg, pork rinds, jalapeno pepper, cream cheese, garlic powder, dried oregano, salt, and onion powder.

3. Blend the mixture until smooth.

4. Then with the help of the scooper make the small poppers.

5. Toss the coconut oil in the instant pot and melt it on sauté mode.

6. Then place the salmon poppers in the instant pot in one layer.

7. Cook the meal for 3 minutes from each side or until it is light brown.

8. Dry the cooked salmon poppers with the help of the paper towels if needed.

Nutrition value/serving: calories 135, fat 8.8, fiber 0.2, carbs 0.8, protein 13.7

Tuna Nutmeg Rolls

Prep time: 20 minutes

Cooking time: 20 minutes

Servings: 4

Ingredients:

- 4 kale leaves
- 10 oz tuna, canned
- ½ white onion, minced
- 1 teaspoon ground coriander
- ½ teaspoon salt
- ½ teaspoon ground paprika
- ¼ teaspoon ground nutmeg
- 2 oz leek, chopped
- 1 teaspoon avocado oil
- 1 cup water, for cooking

Directions:

1. Pour avocado oil in the instant pot.

2. Add chopped leek and minced white onion.

3. Cook the vegetables on sauté mode for 5 minutes.

4. Stir the mixture from time to time with the help of the spatula.

5. Then add tuba, salt, ground coriander, ground paprika, ground nutmeg, and mix up well.

6. Then transfer the mixture in the bowl and clean the instant pot.

7. Pour water and insert the steamer rack in the instant pot.

8. Then fill every kale leaf with tuna mix tuna mixture and roll.

9. Arrange the tuna rolls on the rack and close the lid.

10. Cook the tuna rolls on manual mode (high pressure) for 15 minutes.

11. Then allow the natural pressure release for 10 minutes.

Nutrition value/serving: calories 157, fat 6, fiber 1, carbs 5.3, protein 19.7

Tilapia Sticks

Prep time: 15 minutes

Cooking time: 7 minutes

Servings: 2

Ingredients:

- 8 oz tilapia fillet
- ¼ cup coconut flakes
- 1 egg, beaten
- ¼ teaspoon chili flakes
- ¼ teaspoon ground nutmeg
- 1 tablespoon sesame oil
- 1 cup water, for cooking

Directions:

1. Cut the tilapia fillet into 2 sticks.

2. Then pour water and insert the steamer rack in the instant pot.

3. Line the rack with foil and place the tilapia sticks on it.

4. Close the lid and cook them for 3 minutes on manual mode (high pressure).

5.   When the time is over, make a quick pressure release and open the lid.

6.   Dip the cooked fish sticks in the egg and then coat in the coconut flakes.

7.   Clean the instant pot and remove the steamer rack.

8.   Pour sesame oil in the instant pot and place the tilapia sticks.

9.   Cook them for 1 minute from each side on sauté mode or until the fish sticks are light brown.

Nutrition value/serving: calories 222, fat 13.5, fiber 1, carbs 1.8, protein 24.2

Rangoon Crab Dip

Prep time: 10 minutes

Cooking time: 1.5 hours

Servings: 4

Ingredients:

- 1 teaspoon Erythritol
- 3 tablespoons cream cheese
- 1 tablespoon chives, chopped
- ½ cup whipped cream
- 6 oz crab meat, chopped
- ¼ teaspoon garlic powder

Directions:

1. Place all ingredients in the instant pot and stir well.

2. Close the lid and cook the dip on manual (low pressure) for 1.5 hours.

Nutrition value/serving: calories 109, fat 8, fiber 0, carbs 2.8, protein 6.3

Conclusion

Being a perfect remedy both for instant pot newbies and skilled instant pot individuals this instantaneous pot cookbook elevates your everyday cooking. It makes you look like a professional and also prepare like a pro. Thanks to the Immediate Pot part, this recipe book helps you with preparing straightforward and tasty meals for any kind of budget plan. Satisfy everybody with hearty suppers, nutritious morning meals, sweetest desserts, and fun treats.

No matter if you cook for one or prepare bigger parts-- there's a remedy for any possible cooking scenario. Boost your techniques on just how to prepare in the most reliable way using just your instant pot, this cookbook, and also some patience to learn quick. Handy tips as well as methods are discreetly incorporated right into every recipe to make your household demand brand-new meals time and time again. Vegetarian choices, services for meat-eaters and very pleasing concepts to unify the whole household at the exact same table. Eating in the house is a shared experience, and also it can be so great to satisfy completely at the end of the day. Master your Instantaneous Pot and make the most of this brand-new experience beginning today!

ation can be obtained
q.com
A
110521
00011B/2346